# The "O, MY" in TonsillectOMY & AdenoidectOMY

# How to Prepare Your Child for Surgery

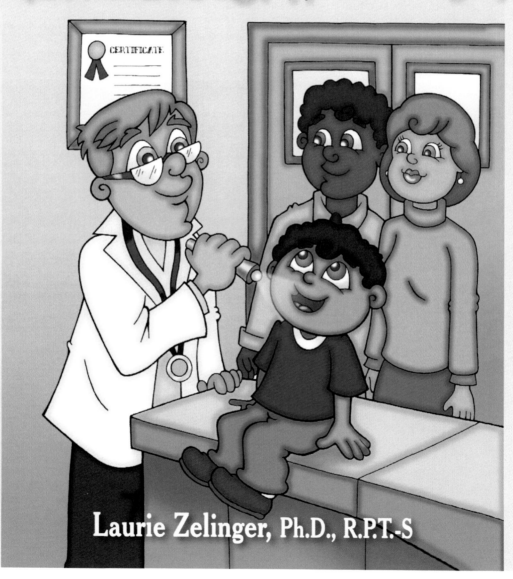

Laurie Zelinger, Ph.D., R.P.T.-S

The "O, my" in tonsillectomy & adenoidectomy : how to prepare your child for surgery, a parent's manual.
Book #3 in the Growing with Love Series
Copyright © 2009 by Laurie Zelinger.

Library of Congress Cataloging-in-Publication Data

Zelinger, Laurie E.
  The "O, my" in tonsillectomy & adenoidectomy : how to prepare your child for surgery, a parent's manual / by Laurie Zelinger.
      p. cm. -- (Growing with love ; book #3)
  Includes bibliographical references.
  ISBN-13: 978-1-932690-74-3 (trade paper : alk. paper)
  ISBN-10: 1-932690-74-3 (trade paper : alk. paper)
  1. Tonsillectomy. 2. Adenoidectomy. 3. Tonsillitis. 4. Children--Surgery. I. Title. II. Title: "O, my" in tonsillectomy and adenoidectomy.
  RF484.5.Z45 2009
  617.5'32--dc22
                                        2008035918

Published by:
Loving Healing Press
5145 Pontiac Trail
Ann Arbor, MI 48105
USA

http://www.LovingHealing.com or
info@LovingHealing.com
Tollfree 888 761 6268
Fax 734 663 6861

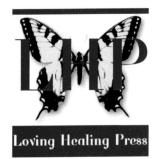

Loving Healing Press

# Table of Contents

Dedicated to
Jordan, Elliot, Perry and David,
my four best reasons for learning how to ease a child
through the difficult times in life.

# Foreword

I have had the pleasure of knowing Dr. Laurie Zelinger through the care of her son. As a caring person involved with children, she brought her clinical insights into the office, especially when discussing her son.

Dr. Zelinger became interested in this project while preparing for her own son's surgery. She has had 'first-hand experience and decided to write to help prepare others for this significant life event. I believe she has addressed parental concerns and the way parents might best interact with their children to prepare them for these procedures.

She deserves a great deal of credit for the way she dealt the needs of her own family, and especially her ability to transform that experience so that others might benefit.

Mark. N. Goldstein, M.D., P.C.
Fellow, American Academy of Otolaryngology
Fellow, American Academy of Pediatrics
Fellow, American College of Surgeons

# Preface

This manual is intended as a guide toward navigating the preparation and surgical process that you and your child are about to undergo. The pronouns and particulars reflect those that pertained to our own situation. Please change them as needed, to reflect your circumstances. If you do not have the luxury of several weeks for preparation, read through this manual in its entirety and select those recommendations that are practical for your lifestyle and time frame, condensing and accelerating the suggestions to fit your schedule.

Dr. Laurie Zelinger
Child Psychologist

# Uh-Oh, Surgery! Making Your Decision

You have just had your consultation with your doctor and he gave you the news. Based on the frequency of your child's sore throats over the past year and other criteria established by the American Academy of Otolaryngology, your doctor is now recommending surgery to remove your child's tonsils. Tonsillectomies and adenoidectomies (T&As) account for the second most common surgical procedure performed on children in the USA (Children's Hospital and Health System, 2008), and are estimated to occur at a frequency of 200,00 to 260,000 per year for children under age 18 (Drake 2007). In fact, T&As account for one-third of all surgeries performed under general anesthesia in the United States.

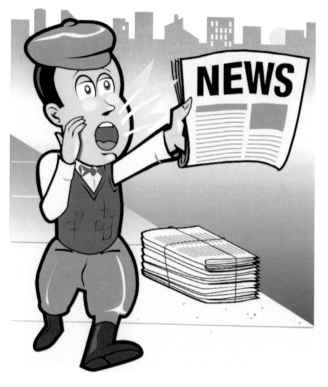

You are now flooded with emotions and information and don't know what to do next. Maybe your child even overheard some of the conversation at the doctor's office. What do you do first? You have an option to schedule surgery on the spot, or to go home and sort things out. My suggestion is to defer any conversation until you and your partner, or other involved person, can speak comfortably and privately. Do not discuss this topic on the car ride home. Children do not need to hear both sides of a situation, or any concerns that you may have. The message that they must get is that you (both) wholeheartedly endorse any decision that you arrive at, and that there is no room for doubt or change of mind.

Never assume that your child is too young to understand what you might discuss. Even if the words are not fully understood, your tone of voice and gestures will convey your feelings. Wait until you are alone to discuss your options. If your child asks what will be happening, reassure him that nothing is happening yet. The doctor visit is over, and now you are going home (or wherever). You might say that Mommy and Daddy and the Ear/Nose/Throat (ENT) doctor are all working together to figure out the best way to help his throat and ears to feel better. This explanation should be enough to quell any immediate concerns. Then, use the next few days to think about the recommendations, and speak with your pediatrician. You may even want to get a second opinion.

Once you have actually scheduled surgery, preparation begins for you and your child. Read everything that you are given about the procedure, until you feel that most of your own questions are answered. Then, and only then, can you begin to prepare your child.

# Phase 1: Introducing the Topic to Your Child

## *1 to 2 Months before Surgery*

You may want to ask your ENT doctor to recommend a child's book for you to read to your youngster. *Your T&A Journey* (2005) and *Good-Bye Tonsils!* (Hatkoff & Hatkoff, 2001) are among such references that share information about the procedure, while *Barney is Best* (Carlstrom, 1994) is suited for a very young child. At some reasonable time before the surgery (several weeks if you have the luxury of time), leave the book within your child's reach to casually investigate. After you have noticed some interest, begin to read it to your youngster for the first time. You

probably will not have a chance to get through the entire story. Every few days, begin to read it over from the beginning, trying to add a paragraph or page at each new reading. The aim is to familiarize your child at his own pace. Stop reading if your child becomes upset. Put it down for a few days and try again later. Whatever amount accomplish at this point is fine, since your goal is just to set the stage for future discussion.

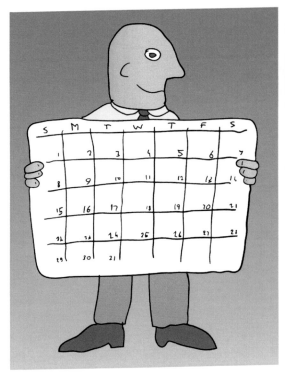

Several weeks before surgery, indicate to your child that one day, but not yet, he will have his tonsils out too, just like the kids in the book you read. Then he will feel better (i.e., not have to be absent from school and be able to sleep better at night). Be specific about the improvement of his particular recurring symptoms.

Your child may ask you what tonsils and adenoids are. You can say something to this effect (see illustration below):

Lots of parts of our bodies have special jobs. Just like our legs are for walking, our nose is for smelling and our tongue is for tasting, our tonsils have a job too. We have two of them way back in our mouth, by our throat. If we open our mouth wide, and look in with a flashlight, it sort of looks like a stage with the lights off before a show. There is a thing hanging down in the middle. It's called a uvula, and it's like a gymnast who is hanging from the ceiling on the stage. If we look to the sides, we'll see a pink bump on each side that looks like the curtain. Those bumps are the tonsils. Their job is to help our body fight sickness and infection by catching germs that come into our body. When the tonsils get full of germs and stop working well, they are not doing their job and we end up getting sick. Lots of times, the doctor will say that if we get rid of sick tonsils, the rest of our body will feel better.

Another part of our body that has a job like the tonsils is called the adenoids. They're behind the stage, so they're too far back to see when we look in our mouth. When the adenoids get sick, they get bigger and take up a lot of room in our mouth. If we have big tonsils and big adenoids, they take up a lot of space and then it's sometimes hard to breathe (Children's Hospital and Health System, 2008). When that happens, we breathe loud in the daytime, and we snore at night.

But if we take out these parts with all the germs in them, we will breathe easier and feel better. Those parts of our body are extra and we don't need them. There are special doctors who know just the right way to take out tonsils, since a gazillion kids need to get rid of theirs. Mommy and daddy called a lot of doctors and found just the right one we liked the best. His name is Dr. ENT, and he will help your mouth and throat get better.

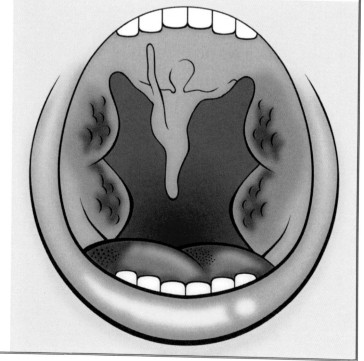

Once you have selected the date and place for surgery, determine where it falls within a time frame that your child can understand. Then use that personal frame of reference in all your future references (e.g., "Your tonsils aren't coming out yet. We will go back to Dr. ENT (after Christmas vacation, after your birthday, when camp starts, etc.) By linking the date of surgery to a personal reference point or major event, your child will be able to gain a more concrete understanding of its occurrence while allaying his fears of an immediate procedure. It will also allow for ample opportunities to bring it up whenever you talk about the holiday, birthday, etc. preceding it. At this point, you should not be giving a drawn-out explanation, but merely a mention of it when the opportunity presents itself.

Within a few weeks, you should be able to ask your child what will happen after Grandma comes to visit (or whatever you have selected as your personal reference point), and his response should become an automatic reply about tonsils, even though he will not yet fully understand the procedure. That's okay at this stage. Use the words, "tonsils" and "adenoids" as often as you can because the more you do, the more you are helping your child to become desensitized to what is likely to be a frightening situation. The more chances he has to talk or to think about it, the more it will inevitably help him to better deal with the procedure. Playing out the procedure using dolls or puppets and a toy medical kit will give your child the opportunity to express her feelings as well as to recognize what questions or worries she may have. The Milton Bradley game "Operation" also introduces the theme of removing and fixing ailing body parts. You may want to make a simple calendar indicating the personal reference point and the date of surgery, so that you can cross off the days as they draw near. This, too, will help your child to feel more control, since children are in a vulnerable situation where only the grown-ups get to call (and, ahem... give) the shots.

# Phase 2: Tackling the Subject

## *What to Tell Your Child 3 to 4 Weeks before Surgery*

About 3 weeks before surgery, your descriptions and references to the procedure will increase. By now you will have made several attempts to read your book to your child. If you have been unsuccessful until now, set aside time when both of you are not distracted and try to read it aloud, even if your child becomes fearful. At this point, read a little more, even through the tears, but keep reassuring him that surgery will not take place until after the personal reference time you have selected. Experts believe that anxiety diminishes as you are able to get mental or physical exposure to the event that is feared. Furthering the discussion is now necessary, and should not be avoided at the child's first sign of discomfort.

Read and talk slowly, and be careful to stay calm when your child protests. Let your child know that you understand what he is feeling. Say something like, "This seems very scary for you." Reassure your child that you will help him to become less afraid. ("Mommy will be there with you the whole time, and will hold you. We will be together. Maybe we'll even bring your teddy bear.")

Do not try to talk your child out of what she is feeling. She is afraid, and telling her not to be will only make her think that you don't understand. Trying to choose the right words to say is not as important as conveying the gentle tone and message that you understand and are trying to do everything you can to help. Let your child know that she can talk about her worries any time she thinks of them. You also want to give the message to all of your children that sick tonsils are not caused by anyone's behavior or anything a child thinks about or wishes. Children can't make someone need a tonsillectomy.

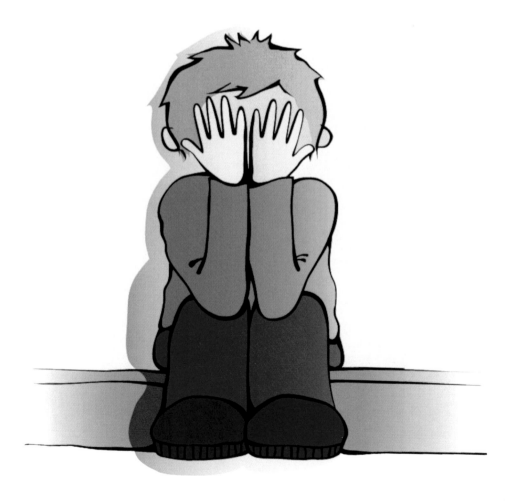

## What to Tell Your Child 2 to 3 Weeks before Surgery

Most people wilt when they hear the words "operation" or "hospital." They have an image in their mind, formed by personal experience, which is frequently exaggerated by "horror" stories or graphic portrayals seen on television. It is your mission to avoid creating these associations for your child. Instead of using the word "operation," describe simply that Dr. ENT will "take out" his tonsils because they have been hurting and you want him to feel better. Rather than using the word "hospital," describe it as Dr. ENT's "other" office at the Day-Op Center. Referring to Dr. ENT by name reduces the mystery and the tendency for your child to invent information. Your child has already had contact with him and has established a frame of reference. An office is a place where children have frequently seen doctors and nurses, and is far less intimidating in one's imagination than a hospital would be.

You may choose to call the operating room a "special room" where the doctor has all the things he needs to fix tonsils, and the term "resting room," because after surgery (in recovery), that is indeed what your child will do. However, if your child is already familiar with other terminology, do not deny the correct terms. The idea is to help your child conceptualize the experience in advance by describing the sequence of events in terms she can understand.

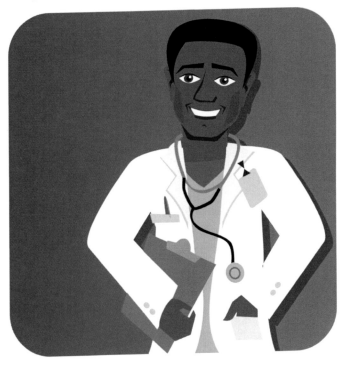

To put this all together as your first explanation to your child, find a time during which you will not be disturbed and when your child is likely to be responsive to you—not while he's watching TV or waiting with bated breath for a playmate to come over. Introduce the topic with reference to the book (which you have now completed together at least once), or by asking what will be happening after (your personal reference point). When your child responds that his tonsils/adenoids will come out, then is your opportunity to take the conversation further.

You might begin by asking your child what he remembers about your prior talks. Then tell him what the day will probably be like. He may stop you several times to talk about something else, or may ask for vivid details about any one procedure. If you don't know the answer to a question, be honest and say so. Tell your child that he asked a great question and you will try to find out the answer. Then make it your business to do so. Even if your child does not seem particularly

attentive, try to describe, even superficially, what he can expect on the day when his tonsils come out. If your child doesn't seem to be giving you his full attention, don't worry. He is probably absorbing some of it and taking in what he is able to handle at the time. This might be a good opportunity to play with dolls and a medical kit, puppets or the Milton-Bradley game "Operation" to acquaint your youngster with the experience.

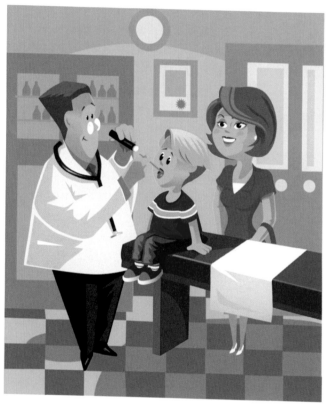

By now, you will also have some idea as to who will be accompanying your child to the medical center. If possible, two adults (with whom he is most comfortable) should be there so that one can attend to the child while the other completes the necessary paperwork. You may also need to take turns later as you sit at your child's bedside, allowing each other to take a break. Additionally, your child may also want someone to sit with him on the ride home as the other one drives. Keep in mind that usually only ONE parent will be allowed into the operating suite. Decide ahead of time whom that will be, if indeed you feel that one of you can be there without getting upset. Then tell some version of the following scenario (see p. 8), and vary it as you see fit for your youngster, personalizing it for your own situation.

## Explaining it all to your 3 to 7-year-old child:

"On the day when your tonsils come out, you will wake up and watch TV like always (or do what you typically do in the morning). Then you will get dressed and can play a little, but we won't have breakfast on that day. After we play, we're going to go in Daddy's car and drive to Dr. ENT's other office at the Day-Op Center. Remember we saw that place already? (Refer to Phase 3 in this manual). When we get there, you and Daddy can play in the playroom while Mommy fills out papers and talks to the lady in the office. When they call our name, we'll go into a little room and a doctor or nurse will look in your ears and nose and mouth and listen to your heart with a stethoscope. Remember what that is? Dr. (your pediatrician's name) wears that around his neck and puts it on your back and chest when he listens to you breathe. The nurse at the Day-Op Center might even take your temperature and blood pressure with that squeezy thing they put around your arm.

"Then we'll go into another office and they will give us different clothes. You can go into a bathroom or dressing room to change. You'll take off your shoes and socks and pants and shirt and underwear. (Some children get very upset at removing their underwear. If you expect that to be the case, speak to the nurse.) They'll give you a costume like a soft pillow case (it's called a gown) that we will tie closed, and maybe even special socks that'll keep you warm and keep you from slipping when you walk. The nurse will also give you a plastic bracelet to wear that will have your name on it and some numbers. And Mommy will have to put on a special costume also. Then we will wait again. We might even see other people in the same kind of gown who are waiting, too. And we'll see doctors and nurses who will be wearing special clothes and even a puffy kind of hat so their hair won't get in the way when they work. Dr. ENT will come out and say hello to us.

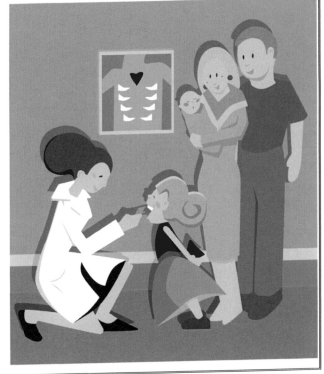

"A little while after that, you might get on a riding toy and drive it right into the "special room" while mommy walks with you. There will be a lot of people in there who are Dr. ENT's helpers, and they will all be wearing the same kind of clothes and maybe a matching cover over their mouth so they can't give us germs if they cough or sneeze. But we'll be able to see their eyes, and when they crinkle, we'll know they are smiling underneath.

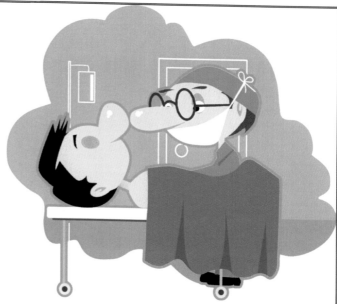

"There will be a lot of silver machines and lights in the 'special room,' everyone will be busy and it will feel cold, since the air conditioner will be on. You'll climb onto a skinny silver table and will lie on your back, or you might sit on Mommy's lap. Mommy will sit on a chair right next to the table and will hold your hand. Then Mommy will give you an astronaut's mask to breathe from that the nurse will hold over your nose and mouth. After a little while it will make you feel dizzy and sleepy. Mommy will stay there until you fall asleep and you will stay asleep until it is all over.

When you wake up, you will be in a different bed and you will see a nurse first, before you see Mommy or Daddy. You'll feel different and your nose and mouth will feel scratchy and will hurt. You'll probably be shivering for a little while. Your stomach might not feel so good either. You might feel like throwing up, but soon you will feel better. Then Mommy and Daddy will come to see you and wait with you while you take a nap. Other children may be taking a nap also in the same room. When you wake up, your arm and hand may have tape on them, and there may be a board under them. There might even be a tube or long straw under your arm and a see-through bag at the other end of the straw which will be hanging on a silver pole right next to your bed. That bag has special medicine and vitamins in it to make you feel better faster.

A different nurse will come to visit you and examine you. She will ask you what you like to drink or what kind of ices you like to eat. You'll feel a little cranky, but if you eat and drink stuff, and make urine ("pee-pee," "sissy"), then you can go home soon. Mommy will help you get your own clothes on and you'll be wheeled to the door in a chair with big wheels on it. Then we will go back home in Daddy's car.

When you get home, you will sleep a lot and you may get mixed up whether it's daytime or nighttime. You will have to stay in bed for a while and can only play quiet games. People might send you cards or presents and everyone will ask how you feel. Your voice will be very low for a few days. Sometimes you will feel good and sometimes you will feel bad. But medicine will help you feel better. You will stay home from school for a lot of days and your voice will probably sound funny for a while. Then, after seven days, you will visit Dr. ENT and he'll look in your mouth. It will not hurt. He will tell you when you can go out and play and when you can eat pizza again and when you can go back to school. By then you will have a lot of energy and will feel like doing everything you used to do. You will be all better and will not get sick so much anymore. You will feel happier and will probably grow a lot and get bigger very fast. And you won't ever have to get your tonsils out again.

# Phase 3: Getting Closer, Getting Ready

## 1 to 2 Weeks to Go

You and your child should be having frequent talks about the surgery by now. Involve him in preparing for those ten long days at home to follow the surgery. Take him shopping with you. Let your child choose his favorite flavor of Jell-o, yogurt, ice cream, pudding, nectar or brand of pastina and creamed cereal. Allow him to select the potatoes that will be cooked for mashed potatoes. Even though he may be long past baby food, many children enjoy permission to eat jarred baby food again. Avoid the tart fruit varieties and all textured foods for the first few days. You'll also need plenty of drinks. Sodas are acceptable if you stir them first to release the bubbles. Be lenient with nutrition rules during the post-operative week. Your goal is to keep your child swallowing anything he can manage. Buy plastic straws and let him help you cut 3 inches off the bottom (shorter straws require less effort for drinking). Pick up interesting cups with different colors, themes, covers, sizes, etc., and plain lollipops without filling. Buy a strip thermometer that can be placed on his forehead, since some children have pain in their ears following this procedure and may not tolerate anything placed in their ear. Your child will probably have difficulty using an oral thermometer now, and the invasive nature of a rectal thermometer may cause added anxiety following surgery.

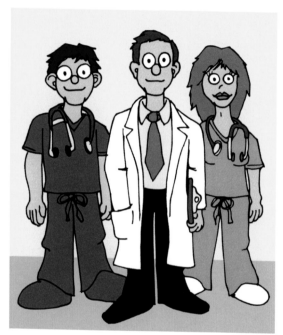

Arrange to visit the medical center where the surgery will take place, either as part of a tour or on your own. Take your child on a leisurely stroll through the waiting room, play room and bathroom. Eat a snack there. Make a phone call or drink from the water fountain. Watch people coming and going.

Stay long enough (15-30 minutes) to help you child form a memory of it and to see enough to talk about. Draw a picture or take a photo of it while you are there, or play "I spy something with my little eye." (To do that, you each take turns locating something in the room and the other person must guess what you are thinking of.) Do not leave until you see that your child is less anxious than when you arrived. You may even use this opportunity to explore the facility if you go there for your lab work one week before surgery.

If you have a good relationship with your dentist, you may want to visit his office to try on the nitrous oxide mask in advance. Let your child feel it, take it on and off, get acquainted with the idea of something over his nose like astronauts use. The actual mask used during surgery will cover his mouth also. However, this is only meant to introduce your child to what she will experience, so there are fewer surprises. You may need to reassure other children in the family that this procedure is not happening to them. Arrange some after school activities for them at the homes of other children and provide a special treat.

Cancel car pool responsibilities and arrange to take time off from work for those important few days after surgery when your child may be feeling miserable. This will remind your child how important she is to you.

## 3 to 7 Days to Go

One week before surgery, your child will need to have necessary and specific lab (blood) work performed. This can be done at an independent laboratory or at the medical center where surgery will be performed. If you expect that the blood test may be particularly upsetting, consider having it done in an independent setting so as not to establish the surgical site as a place to be feared. Ask your pediatrician if he will be requiring any routine blood work also within the near future that could be drawn at the same time, since they often require different tests. This might avoid putting your child through additional blood testing in the pediatrician's office at his next visit.

Go to the library and borrow books that will be saved for the recuperation week. Gather all toys that can be used in bed and store them nearby in one place. Remove the "too active" toys from his view to avoid frustration. You might even move the TV into his room temporarily, buy little gifts or rent new video tapes that can be given when something extra is needed to boost his spirits or break the monotony. Make an audio cassette tape at your next regular reading of a bedtime story. Your child will revel in hearing himself and the story on tape, and you can play it during those post-operative days of bed rest. Your child might appreciate having a bell to ring when he needs you. Set up a daybed and night bed in different rooms if possible, so your child has a change of scenery and cool sheets when he's ready for nighttime sleep. Move a cot into your room for your child, or one into the child's room for you. Use a baby monitor or intercom so he won't have to call you when he needs something.

Schedule a clearance check-up with the pediatrician for the day before surgery.

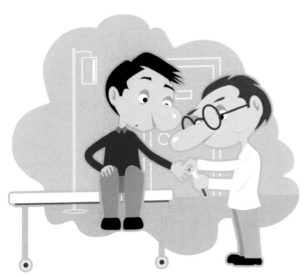

## Counting Down the Days: 3-2-1

Stay calm. Keep your child indoors, and away from other children for a few days before surgery to avoid getting sick (no birthday parties, school or other crowded areas).

Bring your child to the pediatrician for clearance in order to proceed with surgery. If your child is sick, surgery will probably be postponed. In that event, you would describe that being sick means he has germs (i.e., in his throat). Since germs aren't allowed in the "special" room, it is necessary to wait to get his tonsils out until he is better.

Fill all prescriptions for post-surgical medications one day in advance, if possible. Have several medicine dispensers available. Squirting types tend to reduce the need for the child to strain his neck by tilting back to drink from a cup or from a flow-type dispenser. Create a chart to keep track of when you give your child his medications. You may want to ask your child's teacher to send some work home that you can do together toward the end of the week.

# Phase 4: The Day of Surgery — It's Here!

## On the Morning of Surgery

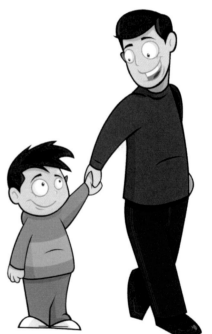

Wake up early enough to eat breakfast, shower and get dressed before waking your child. Take care of the needs of other family members before waking the patient. Change the morning routine slightly so that your child will not come to expect breakfast at the usual time, since he will not be permitted to eat or drink anything. Not even chewing gum.

Pack the following items: an extra front-opening shirt so that your child will not have to strain his neck to get on a pullover; a favorite comforting device (e.g. teddy bear, blanket); a DVD or video tape (there may be a VCR in the recovery room); a distraction for yourself (book, crossword puzzle) enough snacks for a six-hour stay; and prepaid phone card or coins for the pay phone in case cell phones are not permitted. Leave all get-well gifts at home. Your child will be too groggy to enjoy them. Put a blanket, pillow and stomach-sickness bag in the car for the ride home.

## During Surgery

If you are able, accompany your child into the operating room. He may ride a motorized vehicle there and you will walk in and help him to climb onto the table. Be as relaxed and reassuring as possible to your child. He may be frightened and need to focus on you, especially since the rest of the team will be wearing masks and only your voice and face will be recognizable. You might even be allowed to hold him in your lap. Sometimes you are given the option to hold the anesthesia mask over his nose and mouth. As you do so, tell his favorite story in a quiet, calm and slow voice. Continue to make your voice softer as the anesthesia begins to take effect. Be prepared for an agitation phase, when your child may thrash a little under the mask and the pupils of his eyes will become dilated. It may be upsetting to you, but it indicates deepening sedation. Stroke his hair and remind him of your presence. Then leave when you are asked to do so. Expect to wait almost an hour for a T&A procedure. You will be reunited in the recovery room. Often, only one parent at a time is permitted into the recovery room immediately afterward.

## Immediately After Surgery in the Medical Center

Your child will be disoriented. While his eyes may be open, he may not seem to focus or recognize you. Your child may be in a dream-like state even though he is awake. It can be very upsetting to a parent to see a child in an incoherent state and not able to relate to you. This is an after-effect of anesthesia and will wear off with the passing of time. He also may have dried blood around his mouth. If he is able to talk, he may repeat the same questions over and over and may speak at a different rate than usual. He may shiver, cry, sleep or vomit and will probably feel cold. He may want you nearby or to go away or both. Be patient. His behavior will not be predictable, and for a while he may seem like a different child. The constriction of

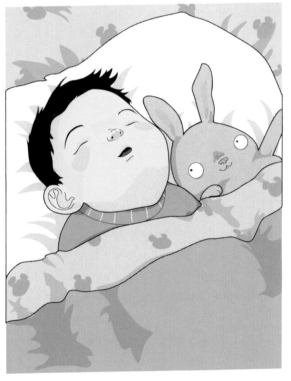

movement from the intravenous tubes will also be frustrating and your child may even succeed in dislodging one. There is little you can do during this difficult period but to wait with your child and to remain as calm as possible. Let him see you. Tell him where he is and that his tonsils are already out. Keep your sentences short and simple, and don't ask questions that require answers. Force fluids, since drinking is essential! You should expect to be in the recovery area for about four hours, most likely sharing space with other families in the same position. Your child's vital signs will be monitored at regular intervals. Fluid intake and output standards (in a bedpan) must be met before you can all go home.

## At Home after Surgery

It is a tremendous relief to be home, but you may worry about recuperation. Keep your physician's phone number handy in the event that you have any concerns. Your phone call will not be an imposition. Write down all of your questions so that you don't forget to ask any. Keep a pen handy to write the answers. Tape your post-operative instruction sheet to a wall near your child's bed, near the phone or on the refrigerator. Also, keep a chart of the times you administer each medication. Acetaminophen (i.e. Tylenol) is generally the only acceptable pain reliever, as ibuprophen and aspirin are contraindicated due to their tendency to cause increased bleeding.

Expect everybody's sleep patterns to be altered. With frequent napping, day and night times may get confused. Some children have nightmares as a result of the anesthesia or the trauma of the actual event. This will improve as recuperation progresses. Nausea may be another effect of general anesthesia, plaguing your child for the next few days unless your physician has prescribed an anti-emetic. Keep a waste basket nearby to avoid the need to run to the bathroom, but cold compresses on the back of the neck sometimes helps. Your child may experience swallowing difficulties. It will be painful, and sometimes when they drink, liquid may move up into the nose as the body readjusts to the changes in the throat. When your child awakens from sleep, there may be some dried blood on her lips. Use a RED washcloth to wipe away (and camouflage) any signs of minor bleeding. Additional pillows should be used to keep her head elevated, and colorful, print pillowcases will detract from stains caused by post-operative oozing. Refrigerate medication to ease in its swallowing. Cold liquids will help to reduce swelling and numb the area.

Allow your child special privileges, since nothing is ordinary about her recent experience.

Restrict traffic in the house to avoid excitement and the tendency to be active too quickly, as well as to avoid contact with others who may be carrying germs. Inform his teacher of the surgery so that the class can make a get-well card. Use your toy medical kit and dolls or puppets to allow your child to act out the recent experience. Play with your child, making sure to do her favorite activities. Take a photo for future reference.

The first three days after surgery are the most difficult, and increased pain is sometimes reported on the fifth day. However, significant improvement will follow over the next few weeks. It is easy to be fooled into thinking that your child is almost better when he shows interest in resuming activities and begins to feel less pain, but do NOT take him out prematurely! Increased activity can result in increased bleeding and may even lengthen the recuperation process. Follow your doctor's advice even if you think that your child is recovering faster than expected. In less than two weeks, your child will be back in school. Since recuperation is a very individual process, comparisons among children should be avoided and existing concerns should be raised only with your doctor.

Over the next few months, you may notice several changes in your child. You may see rapid growth in height and weight, a renewed appetite and interest in food, and a change in the quality of his voice. Resistance to ear, nose and throat infections will improve. Many parents even report improvement in their child's general disposition. While the experience will have undoubtedly been a difficult one for the whole family, children are resilient and bounce back quickly. Their successful journey through pre- and post-surgery will largely be the result of your preparation and effort. They will have you to thank for helping them to cope with what otherwise might have been a terrifying and overwhelming experience. Your child has succeeded in dealing with a difficult situation, learning that he has a foundation to deal with other challenges that come his way.

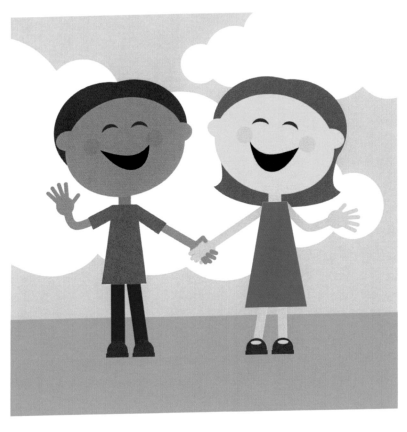

# The Ultimate Preparation List

- ☐ Medical Insurance information
- ☐ Phone numbers for surgeon, pediatrician and pharmacy
- ☐ *Your T&A Journey, Good-Bye Tonsils!* or other recommended book
- ☐ Several medicine dispensers
- ☐ Thermometer (ear or forehead strip)
- ☐ Prescription medications
- ☐ Pain relievers/Acetaminophen
- ☐ Straws
- ☐ Drinks (plenty!)
- ☐ Baby food, pastina, farina, flavored ices, Jell-o, yogurt, pudding, favorite soft foods
- ☐ Bell for child to ring if he needs you
- ☐ Baby monitor or intercom
- ☐ Red washcloths
- ☐ Extra pillows for elevation with printed pillow cases
- ☐ Quiet games/books for recuperation period
- ☐ Video tapes, home made cassette tapes or DVDs
- ☐ Toy medical kit and dolls as patient and doctor
- ☐ "Operation" game by Milton Bradley
- ☐ Set up a day and night bed in different locations
- ☐ Calendar
- ☐ Create a medication chart
- ☐ Make clearance appointment with pediatrician before surgery
- ☐ Make appointment with dentist to see nitrous oxide mask
- ☐ Front opening shirt to wear home after procedure
- ☐ Coins or pre-paid phone card for public telephones at surgical center
- ☐ Car sickness bag for ride home from surgery

# Bibliography

American Academy of Otolaryngology—Head and Neck Surgery. (2008). Fact Sheet: Tonsillitis. Alexandria, VA.

American Academy of Otolaryngology—Head and Neck Surgery. (2008). Fact Sheet: Tonsillectomy Procedures. Alexandria, VA.

American Academy of Otolaryngology—Head and Neck Surgery. (2008). Fact Sheet: Tonsils and Adenoids. Alexandria, VA.

Carlstrom, N. W., & Hale, J. G. (1994). *Barney is best*. New York: HarperCollins.

Children's Hospital and Health System. (2008).Tonsillectomy and Adenoidectomy                    [Online]. http://www.chw.org/display/PPF/DocID/21503/router.asp

Drake, A. & Carr, M. (2007). Tonsillectomy. eMedicine from WebMD [online] http://www.emedicine.com/ent/topic315.htm

Hatkoff, J., Hatkoff, C., & Mets, M. (2001). *Good-bye tonsils!* New York: Viking

Krames, L. A. (2005). *Your T&A journey. Patient information library.* Daly City, CA: Krames Communications.

Stoppler, M. (2005). Does My Child Need a Tonsillectomy? MedicineNet.com [online] http://www.medicinenet.com/script/main/art.asp?articlekey=41583

Tonsillectomy. In Encyclopedia of Surgery: A Guide for Patients and Caregivers. [online]. http://www.surgeryencyclopedia.com/St-Wr/Tonsillectomy.html

Tonsillectomy. (2008, August 3). *The New York Times.* [online]. http://health.nytimes.com/health/guides/surgery/tonsillectomy/overview.html

Wax, M. K. (2004). *Primary care otolaryngology.* Alexandria, VA: American Academy of Otolaryngology--Head and Neck Surgery Foundation.

# Caregiver's Organizer

Current medications:

Allergies:

Health Insurance Information:

| **Pediatrician:** | Address |
|---|---|
| Phone | Fax |

| **Ear/Nose/Throat surgeon**: | Address |
|---|---|
| Phone | Fax |

| **Surgical site:** | Address, |
|---|---|
| Phone | Fax |
| Contact person | |

| **Pharmacy:** | Address |
|---|---|
| Phone | Fax |

| | |
|---|---|
| Date of tour/visit to surgical center: | |
| Date of pre-operation testing: | |
| Date of surgical clearance exam at pediatrician: | |
| DATE of SURGERY: | |
| Post-surgical exam (with Surgeon) | |
| Post-surgical exam (with Pediatrician) | |

Favorite ice cream flavors:

# About the Author

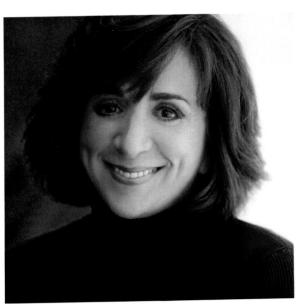

Dr. Laurie Zelinger was born and raised in Queens, New York, and is a successful product of the New York City public school system. She earned her Master's degree and Professional Diploma from Queens College over 30 years ago and later went on to earn a Doctoral degree from Hofstra University. Her interest in children dates back to her days as a babysitter and became the foundation of her later pursuit of school psychology and play therapy. During the course of her professional career, Dr. Zelinger and her psychologist husband, Dr. Fred Zelinger, raised four sons. As parents, they learned first hand the difference between reading about children and living with them.

This book represents the author's actual experience with her son Jordan's tonsillectomy and adenoidectomy, as well as her hope that others will benefit from this information. Her concept of preparing a child for surgery is based upon the premise that information and preparation will reduce anxiety and help families to better manage the experience. Her time lines may also be used as a guide for children undergoing other hospital procedures.

Dr. Zelinger's ongoing devotion to children continues in her role as a school psychologist, private practice licensed psychologist, and registered play therapist. She works and lives on Long Island, New York.

**I'm wishing you a great recovery!**
*Dr. Laurie Zelinger*

## Other Healing Titles You May Like

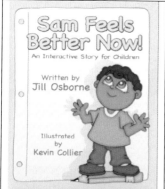

### Sam Feels Better Now! An Interactive Story for Children
### By Jill Osborne, Ed S.

Sam saw something awful and scary! Ms. Carol, a special therapist, will show Sam how to feel better. Children can help Sam feel better too by using drawings, play, and storytelling activities. They will be able to identify and manage their own feelings and difficulties in their lives following a traumatic event, crisis, or grief.

List $24.95 * ISBN 9781932690606

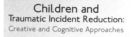
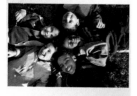
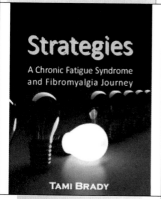

### Strategies: A Chronic Fatigue Syndrome and Fibromyalgia Journey By Tami Brady

I've never been someone who dictates advice, so my book provides worksheets you can develop to tailor your personal responses to symptoms and crises. It is the good, the bad, and the ugly of my personal journey that I share with you. My hope is that you will find solace and renewed hope in my words.

List $17.95 * ISBN 9781932690484

### Children and Traumatic Incident Reduction
### By Marian K. Volkman, CTS, CMF

"This book is a must for any therapist working with kids. Naturally, it focuses on the approach of Traumatic Incident Reduction, but there is a lot of excellent material that will be useful even to the therapist who has never before heard of TIR. The approach is complexly respectful of clients."

—Robert Rich, PhD

List $19.95 * ISBN 9781932690309

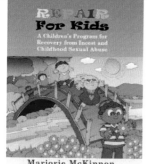

### R.E.P.A.I.R for Kids
### By Marjorie McKinnon

"I found this book to be well thought out and written, and one that would be helpful for any child who has known the pain of sexual abuse. I wish a caring adult had shared this book with my siblings and myself, it would have helped ease our pain and sorrow."

Michael Skinner, musician, child mental health advocate

List $34.95 * ISBN 9781932690576

CPSIA information can be obtained
at www.ICGtesting.com
Printed in the USA
381820LV00013B/81